T

MW01283476

- [ ] Sleep
- [ ] Sleep some more

TO DO LIST

DATE: ____________________

- [ ] Sleep
- [ ] Sleep some more
- [ ]
- [ ]
- [ ]
- [ ]
- [ ]
- [ ]
- [ ]
- [ ]
- [ ]
- [ ]
- [ ]
- [ ]
- [ ]
- [ ]
- [ ]
- [ ]
- [ ]

TO DO LIST

DATE: ______________________

- [ ] Sleep
- [ ] Sleep some more

TO DO LIST

DATE: ______________________

- [ ] Sleep
- [ ] Sleep some more

TO DO LIST

DATE: ____________________

- [ ] Sleep
- [ ] Sleep some more
- [ ]
- [ ]
- [ ]
- [ ]
- [ ]
- [ ]
- [ ]
- [ ]
- [ ]
- [ ]
- [ ]
- [ ]
- [ ]
- [ ]
- [ ]
- [ ]
- [ ]
- [ ]
- [ ]
- [ ]
- [ ]
- [ ]
- [ ]
- [ ]
- [ ]
- [ ]
- [ ]
- [ ]
- [ ]
- [ ]
- [ ]
- [ ]
- [ ]
- [ ]
- [ ]
- [ ]

TO DO LIST

DATE: ______________________

- [ ] Sleep
- [ ] Sleep some more

TO DO LIST

DATE: ______________________

- [ ] Sleep
- [ ] Sleep some more

TO DO LIST

DATE: ______________________

- [ ] Sleep
- [ ] Sleep some more

TO DO LIST

DATE: ____________________

- [ ] Sleep
- [ ] Sleep some more
- [ ]
- [ ]

TO DO LIST

DATE: ____________________

- [ ] Sleep
- [ ] Sleep some more

TO DO LIST

DATE: ______________________

- [ ] Sleep
- [ ] Sleep some more

TO DO LIST

DATE: ____________________

- [ ] Sleep
- [ ] Sleep some more
- [ ]
- [ ]
- [ ]
- [ ]
- [ ]
- [ ]
- [ ]
- [ ]
- [ ]
- [ ]
- [ ]
- [ ]
- [ ]
- [ ]
- [ ]
- [ ]
- [ ]
- [ ]
- [ ]
- [ ]
- [ ]
- [ ]
- [ ]
- [ ]
- [ ]
- [ ]
- [ ]
- [ ]
- [ ]
- [ ]
- [ ]
- [ ]
- [ ]
- [ ]
- [ ]
- [ ]
- [ ]
- [ ]

TO DO LIST

DATE: ______________________

- [ ] Sleep
- [ ] Sleep some more
- [ ]
- [ ]
- [ ]
- [ ]
- [ ]
- [ ]
- [ ]
- [ ]
- [ ]
- [ ]
- [ ]
- [ ]
- [ ]
- [ ]
- [ ]
- [ ]
- [ ]
- [ ]
- [ ]
- [ ]
- [ ]
- [ ]
- [ ]
- [ ]
- [ ]
- [ ]
- [ ]
- [ ]
- [ ]
- [ ]
- [ ]
- [ ]
- [ ]
- [ ]
- [ ]
- [ ]

TO DO LIST

DATE: ____________

- [ ] Sleep
- [ ] Sleep some more
- [ ]
- [ ]

TO DO LIST

DATE: ____________________

- [ ] Sleep
- [ ] Sleep some more
- [ ]
- [ ]
- [ ]
- [ ]
- [ ]
- [ ]
- [ ]
- [ ]
- [ ]
- [ ]
- [ ]
- [ ]
- [ ]
- [ ]
- [ ]
- [ ]
- [ ]

- [ ]
- [ ]
- [ ]
- [ ]
- [ ]
- [ ]
- [ ]
- [ ]
- [ ]
- [ ]
- [ ]
- [ ]
- [ ]
- [ ]
- [ ]
- [ ]
- [ ]
- [ ]
- [ ]

TO DO LIST

DATE: ______________________

- [ ] Sleep
- [ ] Sleep some more

TO DO LIST

DATE: ______

- [ ] Sleep
- [ ] Sleep some more
- [ ]
- [ ]
- [ ]
- [ ]
- [ ]
- [ ]
- [ ]
- [ ]
- [ ]
- [ ]
- [ ]
- [ ]
- [ ]
- [ ]
- [ ]
- [ ]
- [ ]

TO DO LIST

DATE: ______________________

- [ ] Sleep
- [ ] Sleep some more

TO DO LIST

DATE: ____________________

- [ ] Sleep
- [ ] Sleep some more

TO DO LIST

DATE: ______________________

- [ ] Sleep
- [ ] Sleep some more

TO DO LIST

DATE: ____________________

- [ ] Sleep
- [ ] Sleep some more

TO DO LIST

DATE: ____________

- [ ] Sleep
- [ ] Sleep some more
- [ ]
- [ ]
- [ ]
- [ ]
- [ ]
- [ ]
- [ ]
- [ ]
- [ ]
- [ ]
- [ ]
- [ ]
- [ ]
- [ ]
- [ ]
- [ ]
- [ ]

TO DO LIST

DATE: ______________________

- [ ] Sleep
- [ ] Sleep some more

TO DO LIST

DATE: ______

- [ ] Sleep
- [ ] Sleep some more

TO DO LIST

DATE: ______________________

- [ ] Sleep
- [ ] Sleep some more

TO DO LIST

DATE: ______________

- [ ] Sleep
- [ ] Sleep some more

TO DO LIST

DATE: ______________________

- [ ] Sleep
- [ ] Sleep some more

TO DO LIST

DATE: ______

- [ ] Sleep
- [ ] Sleep some more
- [ ]
- [ ]
- [ ]
- [ ]
- [ ]
- [ ]
- [ ]
- [ ]
- [ ]
- [ ]
- [ ]
- [ ]
- [ ]
- [ ]
- [ ]
- [ ]
- [ ]

TO DO LIST

DATE: ______________________

- [ ] Sleep
- [ ] Sleep some more

TO DO LIST

DATE: ______

- [ ] Sleep
- [ ] Sleep some more

TO DO LIST

DATE: ______________________

- [ ] Sleep
- [ ] Sleep some more
- [ ]
- [ ]
- [ ]
- [ ]
- [ ]
- [ ]
- [ ]
- [ ]
- [ ]
- [ ]
- [ ]
- [ ]
- [ ]
- [ ]
- [ ]
- [ ]
- [ ]
- [ ]
- [ ]
- [ ]
- [ ]
- [ ]
- [ ]
- [ ]
- [ ]
- [ ]
- [ ]
- [ ]
- [ ]
- [ ]
- [ ]
- [ ]
- [ ]
- [ ]
- [ ]
- [ ]

TO DO LIST

DATE: ______________________

- [ ] Sleep
- [ ] Sleep some more

TO DO LIST

DATE: ____________________

- [ ] Sleep
- [ ] Sleep some more

TO DO LIST

DATE: ______

- [ ] Sleep
- [ ] Sleep some more

TO DO LIST

DATE: ____________________

- [ ] Sleep
- [ ] Sleep some more
- [ ]
- [ ]
- [ ]
- [ ]
- [ ]
- [ ]
- [ ]
- [ ]
- [ ]
- [ ]
- [ ]
- [ ]
- [ ]
- [ ]
- [ ]
- [ ]
- [ ]

TO DO LIST

DATE: ______________________

- [ ] Sleep
- [ ] Sleep some more

TO DO LIST

DATE: ____________________

- [ ] Sleep
- [ ] Sleep some more
- [ ]
- [ ]
- [ ]
- [ ]
- [ ]
- [ ]
- [ ]
- [ ]
- [ ]
- [ ]
- [ ]
- [ ]
- [ ]
- [ ]
- [ ]
- [ ]
- [ ]
- [ ]
- [ ]
- [ ]
- [ ]
- [ ]
- [ ]
- [ ]
- [ ]
- [ ]
- [ ]
- [ ]
- [ ]
- [ ]
- [ ]
- [ ]
- [ ]
- [ ]
- [ ]
- [ ]

TO DO LIST

DATE: __________

- [ ] Sleep
- [ ] Sleep some more

TO DO LIST

DATE: ______________________

- [ ] Sleep
- [ ] Sleep some more
- [ ]
- [ ]
- [ ]
- [ ]
- [ ]
- [ ]
- [ ]
- [ ]
- [ ]
- [ ]
- [ ]
- [ ]
- [ ]
- [ ]
- [ ]
- [ ]
- [ ]
- [ ]
- [ ]
- [ ]
- [ ]
- [ ]
- [ ]
- [ ]
- [ ]
- [ ]
- [ ]
- [ ]
- [ ]
- [ ]
- [ ]
- [ ]
- [ ]
- [ ]
- [ ]
- [ ]

TO DO LIST

DATE: ______________________

- [ ] Sleep
- [ ] Sleep some more
- [ ]
- [ ]
- [ ]
- [ ]
- [ ]
- [ ]
- [ ]
- [ ]
- [ ]
- [ ]
- [ ]
- [ ]
- [ ]
- [ ]
- [ ]
- [ ]
- [ ]

TO DO LIST

DATE: ____________________

- [ ] Sleep
- [ ] Sleep some more

TO DO LIST

DATE: ______________________

- [ ] Sleep
- [ ] Sleep some more
- [ ]
- [ ]
- [ ]
- [ ]
- [ ]
- [ ]
- [ ]
- [ ]
- [ ]
- [ ]
- [ ]
- [ ]
- [ ]
- [ ]
- [ ]
- [ ]
- [ ]
- [ ]
- [ ]
- [ ]
- [ ]
- [ ]
- [ ]
- [ ]
- [ ]
- [ ]
- [ ]
- [ ]
- [ ]
- [ ]
- [ ]
- [ ]
- [ ]
- [ ]
- [ ]
- [ ]
- [ ]
- [ ]

TO DO LIST

DATE: ______________________

- [ ] Sleep
- [ ] Sleep some more
- [ ]
- [ ]
- [ ]
- [ ]
- [ ]
- [ ]
- [ ]
- [ ]
- [ ]
- [ ]
- [ ]
- [ ]
- [ ]
- [ ]
- [ ]
- [ ]
- [ ]
- [ ]
- [ ]
- [ ]
- [ ]
- [ ]
- [ ]
- [ ]
- [ ]
- [ ]
- [ ]
- [ ]
- [ ]
- [ ]
- [ ]
- [ ]
- [ ]
- [ ]
- [ ]
- [ ]
- [ ]
- [ ]

TO DO LIST

DATE: ____________________

- [ ] Sleep
- [ ] Sleep some more

TO DO LIST

DATE: ______________________

- [ ] Sleep
- [ ] Sleep some more

TO DO LIST

DATE: ____________________

- [ ] Sleep
- [ ] Sleep some more

TO DO LIST

DATE: ____________________

- [ ] Sleep
- [ ] Sleep some more
- [ ]
- [ ]
- [ ]
- [ ]
- [ ]
- [ ]
- [ ]
- [ ]
- [ ]
- [ ]
- [ ]
- [ ]
- [ ]
- [ ]
- [ ]
- [ ]
- [ ]
- [ ]
- [ ]
- [ ]
- [ ]
- [ ]
- [ ]
- [ ]
- [ ]
- [ ]
- [ ]
- [ ]
- [ ]
- [ ]
- [ ]
- [ ]
- [ ]
- [ ]
- [ ]
- [ ]

TO DO LIST

DATE: ____________________

- [ ] Sleep
- [ ] Sleep some more

TO DO LIST

DATE: ____________________

- [ ] Sleep
- [ ] Sleep some more

TO DO LIST

DATE: ____________________

- [ ] Sleep
- [ ] Sleep some more

TO DO LIST

DATE: ______________________

- [ ] Sleep
- [ ] Sleep some more
- [ ]
- [ ]
- [ ]
- [ ]
- [ ]
- [ ]
- [ ]
- [ ]
- [ ]
- [ ]
- [ ]
- [ ]
- [ ]
- [ ]
- [ ]
- [ ]
- [ ]
- [ ]
- [ ]
- [ ]
- [ ]
- [ ]
- [ ]
- [ ]
- [ ]
- [ ]
- [ ]
- [ ]
- [ ]
- [ ]
- [ ]
- [ ]
- [ ]
- [ ]
- [ ]
- [ ]
- [ ]
- [ ]

TO DO LIST

DATE: ______________________

- [ ] Sleep
- [ ] Sleep some more

TO DO LIST

DATE: ____________________

- [ ] Sleep
- [ ] Sleep some more
- [ ]
- [ ]
- [ ]
- [ ]
- [ ]
- [ ]
- [ ]
- [ ]
- [ ]
- [ ]
- [ ]
- [ ]
- [ ]
- [ ]
- [ ]
- [ ]
- [ ]
- [ ]
- [ ]
- [ ]
- [ ]
- [ ]
- [ ]
- [ ]
- [ ]
- [ ]
- [ ]
- [ ]
- [ ]
- [ ]
- [ ]
- [ ]
- [ ]
- [ ]
- [ ]
- [ ]

TO DO LIST

DATE: ______________________

- [ ] Sleep
- [ ] Sleep some more
- [ ]
- [ ]
- [ ]
- [ ]
- [ ]
- [ ]
- [ ]
- [ ]
- [ ]
- [ ]
- [ ]
- [ ]
- [ ]
- [ ]
- [ ]
- [ ]
- [ ]

- [ ]
- [ ]
- [ ]
- [ ]
- [ ]
- [ ]
- [ ]
- [ ]
- [ ]
- [ ]
- [ ]
- [ ]
- [ ]
- [ ]
- [ ]
- [ ]
- [ ]
- [ ]
- [ ]

TO DO LIST

DATE: ____________________

- [ ] Sleep
- [ ] Sleep some more
- [ ]
- [ ]
- [ ]
- [ ]
- [ ]
- [ ]
- [ ]
- [ ]
- [ ]
- [ ]
- [ ]
- [ ]
- [ ]
- [ ]
- [ ]
- [ ]
- [ ]
- [ ]
- [ ]
- [ ]
- [ ]
- [ ]
- [ ]
- [ ]
- [ ]
- [ ]
- [ ]
- [ ]
- [ ]
- [ ]
- [ ]
- [ ]
- [ ]
- [ ]
- [ ]
- [ ]

TO DO LIST

DATE: ______________________

- [ ] Sleep
- [ ] Sleep some more

TO DO LIST

DATE: ____________________

- [ ] Sleep
- [ ] Sleep some more

TO DO LIST

DATE: ____________________

- [ ] Sleep
- [ ] Sleep some more
- [ ]
- [ ]
- [ ]
- [ ]
- [ ]
- [ ]
- [ ]
- [ ]
- [ ]
- [ ]
- [ ]
- [ ]
- [ ]
- [ ]
- [ ]
- [ ]
- [ ]

- [ ]
- [ ]
- [ ]
- [ ]
- [ ]
- [ ]
- [ ]
- [ ]
- [ ]
- [ ]
- [ ]
- [ ]
- [ ]
- [ ]
- [ ]
- [ ]
- [ ]
- [ ]
- [ ]

TO DO LIST

DATE: ______________________

- [ ] Sleep
- [ ] Sleep some more
- [ ]
- [ ]
- [ ]
- [ ]
- [ ]
- [ ]
- [ ]
- [ ]
- [ ]
- [ ]
- [ ]
- [ ]
- [ ]
- [ ]
- [ ]
- [ ]
- [ ]
- [ ]
- [ ]
- [ ]
- [ ]
- [ ]
- [ ]
- [ ]
- [ ]
- [ ]
- [ ]
- [ ]
- [ ]
- [ ]
- [ ]
- [ ]
- [ ]
- [ ]
- [ ]
- [ ]

TO DO LIST

DATE: ____________________

- [ ] Sleep
- [ ] Sleep some more

TO DO LIST

DATE: ____________

- [ ] Sleep
- [ ] Sleep some more
- [ ]
- [ ]
- [ ]
- [ ]
- [ ]
- [ ]
- [ ]
- [ ]
- [ ]
- [ ]
- [ ]
- [ ]
- [ ]
- [ ]
- [ ]
- [ ]
- [ ]
- [ ]
- [ ]
- [ ]
- [ ]
- [ ]
- [ ]
- [ ]
- [ ]
- [ ]
- [ ]
- [ ]
- [ ]
- [ ]
- [ ]
- [ ]
- [ ]
- [ ]
- [ ]
- [ ]

TO DO LIST

DATE: ____________________

- [ ] Sleep
- [ ] Sleep some more

TO DO LIST

DATE: ______________________

- [ ] Sleep
- [ ] Sleep some more

TO DO LIST

DATE: ____________________

- [ ] Sleep
- [ ] Sleep some more

TO DO LIST

DATE: ______________________

- [ ] Sleep
- [ ] Sleep some more

TO DO LIST

DATE: ____________________

- [ ] Sleep
- [ ] Sleep some more

TO DO LIST

DATE: ______________________

- [ ] Sleep
- [ ] Sleep some more
- [ ]
- [ ]
- [ ]
- [ ]
- [ ]
- [ ]
- [ ]
- [ ]
- [ ]
- [ ]
- [ ]
- [ ]
- [ ]
- [ ]
- [ ]
- [ ]
- [ ]
- [ ]
- [ ]
- [ ]
- [ ]
- [ ]
- [ ]
- [ ]
- [ ]
- [ ]
- [ ]
- [ ]
- [ ]
- [ ]
- [ ]
- [ ]
- [ ]
- [ ]
- [ ]
- [ ]

TO DO LIST

DATE: ______________________

- [ ] Sleep
- [ ] Sleep some more

TO DO LIST

DATE: ______________________

- [ ] Sleep
- [ ] Sleep some more

TO DO LIST

DATE: ____________________

- [ ] Sleep
- [ ] Sleep some more
- [ ]
- [ ]
- [ ]
- [ ]
- [ ]
- [ ]
- [ ]
- [ ]
- [ ]
- [ ]
- [ ]
- [ ]
- [ ]
- [ ]
- [ ]
- [ ]
- [ ]
- [ ]
- [ ]
- [ ]
- [ ]
- [ ]
- [ ]
- [ ]
- [ ]
- [ ]
- [ ]
- [ ]
- [ ]
- [ ]
- [ ]
- [ ]
- [ ]
- [ ]
- [ ]
- [ ]

TO DO LIST

DATE: ____________________

- [ ] Sleep
- [ ] Sleep some more

TO DO LIST

DATE: ______________________

- [ ] Sleep
- [ ] Sleep some more
- [ ]
- [ ]
- [ ]
- [ ]
- [ ]
- [ ]
- [ ]
- [ ]
- [ ]
- [ ]
- [ ]
- [ ]
- [ ]
- [ ]
- [ ]
- [ ]
- [ ]
- [ ]
- [ ]
- [ ]
- [ ]
- [ ]
- [ ]
- [ ]
- [ ]
- [ ]
- [ ]
- [ ]
- [ ]
- [ ]
- [ ]
- [ ]
- [ ]
- [ ]
- [ ]
- [ ]

TO DO LIST

DATE: ______________________

- [ ] Sleep
- [ ] Sleep some more

TO DO LIST

DATE: ____________________

- [ ] Sleep
- [ ] Sleep some more

TO DO LIST

DATE: ____________________

- [ ] Sleep
- [ ] Sleep some more
- [ ]
- [ ]
- [ ]
- [ ]
- [ ]
- [ ]
- [ ]
- [ ]
- [ ]
- [ ]
- [ ]
- [ ]
- [ ]
- [ ]
- [ ]
- [ ]
- [ ]

- [ ]
- [ ]
- [ ]
- [ ]
- [ ]
- [ ]
- [ ]
- [ ]
- [ ]
- [ ]
- [ ]
- [ ]
- [ ]
- [ ]
- [ ]
- [ ]
- [ ]
- [ ]
- [ ]

TO DO LIST

DATE: ____________________

- [ ] Sleep
- [ ] Sleep some more
- [ ]
- [ ]
- [ ]
- [ ]
- [ ]
- [ ]
- [ ]
- [ ]
- [ ]
- [ ]
- [ ]
- [ ]
- [ ]
- [ ]
- [ ]
- [ ]
- [ ]
- [ ]
- [ ]
- [ ]
- [ ]
- [ ]
- [ ]
- [ ]
- [ ]
- [ ]
- [ ]
- [ ]
- [ ]
- [ ]
- [ ]
- [ ]
- [ ]
- [ ]
- [ ]
- [ ]

TO DO LIST

DATE: ____________________

- [ ] Sleep
- [ ] Sleep some more

TO DO LIST

DATE: ______________________

- [ ] Sleep
- [ ] Sleep some more
- [ ]
- [ ]
- [ ]
- [ ]
- [ ]
- [ ]
- [ ]
- [ ]
- [ ]
- [ ]
- [ ]
- [ ]
- [ ]
- [ ]
- [ ]
- [ ]
- [ ]
- [ ]
- [ ]
- [ ]
- [ ]
- [ ]
- [ ]
- [ ]
- [ ]
- [ ]
- [ ]
- [ ]
- [ ]
- [ ]
- [ ]
- [ ]
- [ ]
- [ ]
- [ ]
- [ ]
- [ ]
- [ ]

TO DO LIST

DATE: ______________________

- [ ] Sleep
- [ ] Sleep some more

TO DO LIST

DATE: ______________________

- [ ] Sleep
- [ ] Sleep some more
- [ ]
- [ ]
- [ ]
- [ ]
- [ ]
- [ ]
- [ ]
- [ ]
- [ ]
- [ ]
- [ ]
- [ ]
- [ ]
- [ ]
- [ ]
- [ ]
- [ ]

- [ ]
- [ ]
- [ ]
- [ ]
- [ ]
- [ ]
- [ ]
- [ ]
- [ ]
- [ ]
- [ ]
- [ ]
- [ ]
- [ ]
- [ ]
- [ ]
- [ ]
- [ ]
- [ ]

TO DO LIST

DATE: ______

- [ ] Sleep
- [ ] Sleep some more
- [ ]
- [ ]
- [ ]
- [ ]
- [ ]
- [ ]
- [ ]
- [ ]
- [ ]
- [ ]
- [ ]
- [ ]
- [ ]
- [ ]
- [ ]
- [ ]
- [ ]

- [ ]
- [ ]
- [ ]
- [ ]
- [ ]
- [ ]
- [ ]
- [ ]
- [ ]
- [ ]
- [ ]
- [ ]
- [ ]
- [ ]
- [ ]
- [ ]
- [ ]
- [ ]
- [ ]

TO DO LIST

DATE: ______________________

- [ ] Sleep
- [ ] Sleep some more
- [ ]
- [ ]
- [ ]
- [ ]
- [ ]
- [ ]
- [ ]
- [ ]
- [ ]
- [ ]
- [ ]
- [ ]
- [ ]
- [ ]
- [ ]
- [ ]
- [ ]
- [ ]
- [ ]
- [ ]
- [ ]
- [ ]
- [ ]
- [ ]
- [ ]
- [ ]
- [ ]
- [ ]
- [ ]
- [ ]
- [ ]
- [ ]
- [ ]
- [ ]
- [ ]
- [ ]

TO DO LIST

DATE: ______________________

- [ ] Sleep
- [ ] Sleep some more
- [ ]
- [ ]
- [ ]
- [ ]
- [ ]
- [ ]
- [ ]
- [ ]
- [ ]
- [ ]
- [ ]
- [ ]
- [ ]
- [ ]
- [ ]
- [ ]
- [ ]
- [ ]
- [ ]
- [ ]
- [ ]
- [ ]
- [ ]
- [ ]
- [ ]
- [ ]
- [ ]
- [ ]
- [ ]
- [ ]
- [ ]
- [ ]
- [ ]
- [ ]
- [ ]
- [ ]

TO DO LIST

DATE: ____________________

- [ ] Sleep
- [ ] Sleep some more

TO DO LIST

DATE: ________________

- [ ] Sleep
- [ ] Sleep some more

TO DO LIST

DATE: ______

- [ ] Sleep
- [ ] Sleep some more
- [ ]
- [ ]

TO DO LIST

DATE: ____________________

- [ ] Sleep
- [ ] Sleep some more
- [ ]
- [ ]
- [ ]
- [ ]
- [ ]
- [ ]
- [ ]
- [ ]
- [ ]
- [ ]
- [ ]
- [ ]
- [ ]
- [ ]
- [ ]
- [ ]
- [ ]
- [ ]
- [ ]
- [ ]
- [ ]
- [ ]
- [ ]
- [ ]
- [ ]
- [ ]
- [ ]
- [ ]
- [ ]
- [ ]
- [ ]
- [ ]
- [ ]
- [ ]
- [ ]
- [ ]

TO DO LIST

DATE: ______________________

- [ ] Sleep
- [ ] Sleep some more

TO DO LIST

DATE: ______________________

- [ ] Sleep
- [ ] Sleep some more
- [ ]
- [ ]
- [ ]
- [ ]
- [ ]
- [ ]
- [ ]
- [ ]
- [ ]
- [ ]
- [ ]
- [ ]
- [ ]
- [ ]
- [ ]
- [ ]

- [ ]
- [ ]
- [ ]
- [ ]
- [ ]
- [ ]
- [ ]
- [ ]
- [ ]
- [ ]
- [ ]
- [ ]
- [ ]
- [ ]
- [ ]
- [ ]
- [ ]
- [ ]

TO DO LIST

DATE: ______________________

- [ ] Sleep
- [ ] Sleep some more
- [ ]
- [ ]
- [ ]
- [ ]
- [ ]
- [ ]
- [ ]
- [ ]
- [ ]
- [ ]
- [ ]
- [ ]
- [ ]
- [ ]
- [ ]
- [ ]
- [ ]

- [ ]
- [ ]
- [ ]
- [ ]
- [ ]
- [ ]
- [ ]
- [ ]
- [ ]
- [ ]
- [ ]
- [ ]
- [ ]
- [ ]
- [ ]
- [ ]
- [ ]
- [ ]
- [ ]

TO DO LIST

DATE: ____________________

- [ ] Sleep
- [ ] Sleep some more

TO DO LIST

DATE: ______________________

- [ ] Sleep
- [ ] Sleep some more
- [ ]
- [ ]
- [ ]
- [ ]
- [ ]
- [ ]
- [ ]
- [ ]
- [ ]
- [ ]
- [ ]
- [ ]
- [ ]
- [ ]
- [ ]
- [ ]
- [ ]

- [ ]
- [ ]
- [ ]
- [ ]
- [ ]
- [ ]
- [ ]
- [ ]
- [ ]
- [ ]
- [ ]
- [ ]
- [ ]
- [ ]
- [ ]
- [ ]
- [ ]
- [ ]
- [ ]

TO DO LIST

DATE: ______________________

- [ ] Sleep
- [ ] Sleep some more

TO DO LIST

DATE: ____________

- [ ] Sleep
- [ ] Sleep some more
- [ ]
- [ ]
- [ ]
- [ ]
- [ ]
- [ ]
- [ ]
- [ ]
- [ ]
- [ ]
- [ ]
- [ ]
- [ ]
- [ ]
- [ ]
- [ ]
- [ ]

TO DO LIST

DATE: ____________________

- [ ] Sleep
- [ ] Sleep some more
- [ ]
- [ ]
- [ ]
- [ ]
- [ ]
- [ ]
- [ ]
- [ ]
- [ ]
- [ ]
- [ ]
- [ ]
- [ ]
- [ ]
- [ ]
- [ ]
- [ ]

- [ ]
- [ ]
- [ ]
- [ ]
- [ ]
- [ ]
- [ ]
- [ ]
- [ ]
- [ ]
- [ ]
- [ ]
- [ ]
- [ ]
- [ ]
- [ ]
- [ ]
- [ ]
- [ ]

TO DO LIST

DATE: ______________________

- [ ] Sleep
- [ ] Sleep some more

TO DO LIST

DATE: ____________________

- [ ] Sleep
- [ ] Sleep some more
- [ ]
- [ ]
- [ ]
- [ ]
- [ ]
- [ ]
- [ ]
- [ ]
- [ ]
- [ ]
- [ ]
- [ ]
- [ ]
- [ ]
- [ ]
- [ ]
- [ ]
- [ ]
- [ ]
- [ ]
- [ ]
- [ ]
- [ ]
- [ ]
- [ ]
- [ ]
- [ ]
- [ ]
- [ ]
- [ ]
- [ ]
- [ ]
- [ ]
- [ ]
- [ ]
- [ ]

TO DO LIST

DATE: ____________________

- [ ] Sleep
- [ ] Sleep some more
- [ ]
- [ ]
- [ ]
- [ ]
- [ ]
- [ ]
- [ ]
- [ ]
- [ ]
- [ ]
- [ ]
- [ ]
- [ ]
- [ ]
- [ ]
- [ ]
- [ ]
- [ ]
- [ ]
- [ ]
- [ ]
- [ ]
- [ ]
- [ ]
- [ ]
- [ ]
- [ ]
- [ ]
- [ ]
- [ ]
- [ ]
- [ ]
- [ ]
- [ ]
- [ ]
- [ ]

TO DO LIST

DATE: ______________________

- [ ] Sleep
- [ ] Sleep some more
- [ ]
- [ ]
- [ ]
- [ ]
- [ ]
- [ ]
- [ ]
- [ ]
- [ ]
- [ ]
- [ ]
- [ ]
- [ ]
- [ ]
- [ ]
- [ ]
- [ ]

- [ ]
- [ ]
- [ ]
- [ ]
- [ ]
- [ ]
- [ ]
- [ ]
- [ ]
- [ ]
- [ ]
- [ ]
- [ ]
- [ ]
- [ ]
- [ ]
- [ ]
- [ ]
- [ ]

TO DO LIST

DATE: ____________________

- [ ] Sleep
- [ ] Sleep some more
- [ ]
- [ ]
- [ ]
- [ ]
- [ ]
- [ ]
- [ ]
- [ ]
- [ ]
- [ ]
- [ ]
- [ ]
- [ ]
- [ ]
- [ ]
- [ ]
- [ ]

- [ ]
- [ ]
- [ ]
- [ ]
- [ ]
- [ ]
- [ ]
- [ ]
- [ ]
- [ ]
- [ ]
- [ ]
- [ ]
- [ ]
- [ ]
- [ ]
- [ ]
- [ ]
- [ ]

TO DO LIST

DATE: ______________________

- [ ] Sleep
- [ ] Sleep some more

TO DO LIST

DATE: ____________________

- [ ] Sleep
- [ ] Sleep some more
- [ ]
- [ ]
- [ ]
- [ ]
- [ ]
- [ ]
- [ ]
- [ ]
- [ ]
- [ ]
- [ ]
- [ ]
- [ ]
- [ ]
- [ ]
- [ ]
- [ ]
- [ ]
- [ ]
- [ ]
- [ ]
- [ ]
- [ ]
- [ ]
- [ ]
- [ ]
- [ ]
- [ ]
- [ ]
- [ ]
- [ ]
- [ ]
- [ ]
- [ ]
- [ ]
- [ ]
- [ ]
- [ ]

TO DO LIST

DATE: ______________________

- [ ] Sleep
- [ ] Sleep some more
- [ ]
- [ ]
- [ ]
- [ ]
- [ ]
- [ ]
- [ ]
- [ ]
- [ ]
- [ ]
- [ ]
- [ ]
- [ ]
- [ ]
- [ ]
- [ ]
- [ ]
- [ ]
- [ ]
- [ ]
- [ ]
- [ ]
- [ ]
- [ ]
- [ ]
- [ ]
- [ ]
- [ ]
- [ ]
- [ ]
- [ ]
- [ ]
- [ ]
- [ ]
- [ ]
- [ ]

TO DO LIST

DATE: ____________________

- [ ] Sleep
- [ ] Sleep some more

TO DO LIST

DATE: ____________________

- [ ] Sleep
- [ ] Sleep some more
- [ ]
- [ ]
- [ ]
- [ ]
- [ ]
- [ ]
- [ ]
- [ ]
- [ ]
- [ ]
- [ ]
- [ ]
- [ ]
- [ ]
- [ ]
- [ ]
- [ ]
- [ ]
- [ ]
- [ ]
- [ ]
- [ ]
- [ ]
- [ ]
- [ ]
- [ ]
- [ ]
- [ ]
- [ ]
- [ ]
- [ ]
- [ ]
- [ ]
- [ ]
- [ ]
- [ ]

TO DO LIST

DATE: ____________

- [ ] Sleep
- [ ] Sleep some more

TO DO LIST

DATE: ______________________

- [ ] Sleep
- [ ] Sleep some more
- [ ]
- [ ]
- [ ]
- [ ]
- [ ]
- [ ]
- [ ]
- [ ]
- [ ]
- [ ]
- [ ]
- [ ]
- [ ]
- [ ]
- [ ]
- [ ]
- [ ]
- [ ]
- [ ]
- [ ]
- [ ]
- [ ]
- [ ]
- [ ]
- [ ]
- [ ]
- [ ]
- [ ]
- [ ]
- [ ]
- [ ]
- [ ]
- [ ]
- [ ]
- [ ]
- [ ]

TO DO LIST

DATE: ____________________

- [ ] Sleep
- [ ] Sleep some more
- [ ]
- [ ]
- [ ]
- [ ]
- [ ]
- [ ]
- [ ]
- [ ]
- [ ]
- [ ]
- [ ]
- [ ]
- [ ]
- [ ]
- [ ]
- [ ]
- [ ]
- [ ]
- [ ]
- [ ]
- [ ]
- [ ]
- [ ]
- [ ]
- [ ]
- [ ]
- [ ]
- [ ]
- [ ]
- [ ]
- [ ]
- [ ]
- [ ]
- [ ]
- [ ]
- [ ]

TO DO LIST

DATE: ________________

- [ ] Sleep
- [ ] Sleep some more

TO DO LIST

DATE: ______________________

- [ ] Sleep
- [ ] Sleep some more

Made in United States
North Haven, CT
13 March 2023

33868446R00061